A Diabetes Patient's Guide

Managing and Living with Diabetes

George G. Bissett

Disclaimer

Table of Contents

About the book

Living with diabetes can be a trying experience, but it is entirely possible to lead a full and healthy life with the disease, provided it is managed properly and adequate care is received. Diabetes is a long-term disorder that alters the way in which the body processes sugar, also known as glucose, that is found in the blood. Diabetes can be divided into two primary categories: type 1 and type 2.

Insulin, a hormone that plays a role in maintaining normal levels of blood sugar, cannot be produced by people who have type 1 diabetes. Because of this, in order to control their condition, they will need to either inject themselves with insulin or utilize an insulin pump.

Introduction

Samantha had always been an active and healthy person. She enjoyed running, hiking, and playing sports with her friends. But when she was diagnosed with diabetes, she felt like her whole world was turned upside down.

At first, she was overwhelmed by the amount of information she had to learn about managing her condition. She had to monitor her blood sugar levels, take insulin injections, and make careful choices about the foods she ate. It was a lot to handle, and she felt frustrated and scared.

But with the help of her family and healthcare team, Samantha gradually started to get a handle on her diabetes. She learned how to count carbohydrates, plan meals, and adjust her insulin doses. She also found new ways to stay active, like taking up swimming and biking.

Over time, Samantha realized that living with diabetes didn't have to hold her back. She was still able to do all the things she loved, and she even started to feel healthier and more energetic than she had in a long time. She found a support group for people with diabetes, and made new friends who understood what she was going through.

Samantha learned that managing her diabetes was an ongoing process, but she was up for the challenge. She continued to take care of herself, and with the support of her loved ones, she was able to live a happy, healthy life with diabetes.

Chapter One

What really is diabetes?

Diabetes is a condition that lasts for a long time and alters the way in which the body processes glucose, or blood sugar. When glucose is not digested in an appropriate manner, this can result in a variety of health concerns because glucose is the primary source of fuel for the cells in the body. Diabetes can be divided into two primary categories: type 1 and type 2.

Type 1 diabetes, also known as juvenile diabetes or insulin-dependent diabetes, is a form of diabetes that develops when the immune system of the body attacks and destroys the cells in the pancreas that are responsible for producing insulin. Other names for this form of diabetes include insulin-dependent diabetes and juvenile diabetes. Because of this, there is an insufficient amount of insulin in the body, which leads to the body being unable to digest glucose in an appropriate manner. In order to keep their blood sugar levels under control, people who have type 1 diabetes have to either inject themselves with insulin or utilize an insulin pump.

Diabetes type 2, also known as adult-onset diabetes or non-insulin-dependent diabetes, is a form of the disease that develops when the body develops a resistance to the effects of insulin or when the pancreas is unable to produce enough insulin to keep up with the demands of the body. Type 2 diabetes can be prevented by maintaining a healthy weight and exercising regularly. People who have type 2 diabetes may be able to keep their blood sugar levels under control by following a nutritious diet and engaging in regular physical activity; nevertheless, the majority of these people may also need to take medication or insulin in order to maintain their blood sugar levels.

If treatment is not received, either form of diabetes can result in major problems for the patient's health, including cardiovascular disease, nerve damage, and renal disease. Diabetes, on the other hand, does not preclude a person from leading a healthy and active life if it is properly managed and treated.

"Diabetes is a challenge, but it is not a sentence. It is a disease that can be managed and controlled, and it does not have to define who you are or limit what you can achieve."

Life is not over because you have diabetes. Make the most of what you have, be grateful."

Chapter Two

Types of Diabetes

Diabetes can take many forms.

Diabetes can be divided into two primary categories: type 1 and type 2.

Insulin, a hormone that works to help regulate blood sugar levels, is not produced in sufficient quantities when a person has type 1 diabetes. This form of diabetes is typically diagnosed in children and young adults, and it requires the administration of insulin injections on a consistent basis in order to maintain normal levels of blood sugar. Insulin is either ineffectively used by the body or insulin production is insufficient in those with type 2 diabetes. Adults are most likely to be diagnosed with this form of diabetes, which is frequently linked to being overweight and leading a sedentary lifestyle. It is usually manageable by maintaining a balanced diet and engaging in regular physical activity; however, some people may need to take medication in order to keep their blood sugar levels under control.

"You are stronger than your diabetes.
You have the power to manage it and
live a healthy, fulfilling life."
"One small step at a time, you can make
a big difference in managing your
diabetes and improving your overall
health."

Chapter Three

What are the signs that someone might have diabetes?

Diabetes is characterized by a variety of symptoms that might be experienced by a person who may or may not have the condition. These symptoms could include the following:

- An increase in thirst and an increase in the frequency with which you have to urinate are both signs that your blood sugar levels are too high. The body tries to rid itself of the excess sugar by eliminating it through urine. Because of this, a person may have feelings of thirst because their body is losing fluids. Because of this, a person who has diabetes may need to urinate more frequently.

- Hunger is a symptom that a person may have if they have high blood sugar levels, even if they have recently consumed a meal.

- Fatigue can be caused by high blood sugar levels because they can inhibit the body's ability to use glucose as a source of energy. This can lead to feelings of exhaustion.

- Vision impairments High blood sugar levels can cause fluid to build up in the lens of the eye, which can contribute to vision impairments such as blurred vision.

- High blood sugar levels can impede the body's capacity to recover correctly, which can result in a delay in the healing process for cuts and wounds.

- Skin that is dry and flaky might be a symptom of having high blood sugar levels.

- Tingling or numbness in the hands and feet High blood sugar levels can cause nerve injury, which can result in tingling or numbness in the hands and feet.

- Infections more frequently High blood sugar levels can impair the body's immune system, making a person more susceptible to infections. This makes people with diabetes more likely to get sick.

It is essential to keep in mind that some individuals who have diabetes may not have any symptoms at all, particularly in the earlier stages of the condition. Even if you don't think you have diabetes, you should still get checked and screened for it on a regular basis, even if you don't have any symptoms.

"You are not alone on this journey. Reach out to friends, family, and healthcare professionals for support and guidance."

Chapter Four

Diabetes's Root Causes

There are various different varieties of diabetes, but type 1 diabetes and type 2 diabetes are the most frequent forms.

<u>Diabetes type 1</u> is an autoimmune disease that develops when the immune system of the body attacks and destroys the cells in the pancreas that produce insulin. Insulin is a hormone that controls how much blood sugar is in the body. Insulin injections or the use of an insulin pump are the primary forms of treatment for this kind of diabetes, which is typically diagnosed in children and young people.

<u>Diabetes type 2</u> is a metabolic disorder that manifests itself either when the body develops a resistance to the effects of insulin or when the pancreas is unable to produce enough insulin to maintain blood sugar levels within a normal range. Both of these conditions can lead to the development of diabetes type 2. A diagnosis of type 2 diabetes is typically made in adults, and the condition is frequently linked to being overweight or obese, leading a sedentary lifestyle, and having a history of the disease in one's family. It is often treated with a mix of modifications to one's lifestyle (such as one's diet and level of physical activity) and medication.

Prediabetes is a condition that develops when a person's blood sugar levels are higher than normal but are not high enough for them to be diagnosed with diabetes. Other types of diabetes include gestational diabetes, which manifests itself during pregnancy, and type 2 diabetes.

If unchecked, diabetes of either type 1 or type 2 can result in a number of major health consequences, including heart disease, stroke, kidney disease, nerve damage, and blindness.

"Be proud of yourself for making an effort to manage your diabetes and improve your health. Every small step counts."

Chapter Five

Diabetes Predisposing Factors and Risk Factors

There are a number of factors that increase one's likelihood of having diabetes, including the following:

Age: The chance of acquiring diabetes is proportional to a person's age, and this risk rises with age.

Family history: If diabetes runs in your family, there is a greater chance that you will develop the condition yourself.

Obesity: The risk of acquiring diabetes is significantly increased in individuals who are obese or overweight.

Inactivity: There is a correlation between a lack of physical activity and an increased risk of acquiring diabetes.

Unhealthy diet: A diet that is high in refined carbohydrates and unhealthy fats is associated with an increased risk of acquiring diabetes.

High blood pressure: Your chance of acquiring diabetes is increased if you have high blood pressure.

High levels of cholesterol: Having high levels of cholesterol makes you more likely to acquire diabetes.

History of gestational diabetes: If you have a history of having diabetes during pregnancy (also known as gestational diabetes), you are at an elevated risk of acquiring diabetes at a later point in your life.

Women who have polycystic ovarian syndrome (PCOS) have a higher chance of acquiring diabetes than other women.

Prediabetes: If you have prediabetes, you have an increased chance of acquiring type 2 diabetes in the future. The condition known as prediabetes occurs when a person's blood sugar levels are higher than usual but are not yet high enough to be diagnosed with diabetes.

It is essential to keep in mind that some of these risk factors, such as age and genetics, are immutable. Age and family history are two examples. However, you can take steps to manage other risk factors, such as maintaining a healthy weight, getting regular physical activity, and eating a healthy diet, in order to lower your risk of developing diabetes. These steps include maintaining a healthy weight.

"With determination and perseverance, you can manage your diabetes and live a healthy, fulfilling life."

"Remember, every day is a chance to make positive changes for your health and well-being."

Chapter six

Diagnosing Diabetes

Diabetes can be diagnosed in a number of different ways, including the following:

Test of fasting blood sugar: This test analyzes your blood sugar after you have not consumed any meals for at least 8 hours before doing the test. Diabetes may be present when the level of glucose in the blood while fasting is 126 milligrams per deciliter (mg/dL) or greater.

The oral glucose tolerance test, also known as the OGTT, requires participants to consume a sweet solution and then have their blood sugar levels monitored at various intervals throughout the test. Diabetes may be present if the blood sugar level is over 200 mg/dL after being monitored for two hours.

A1C test: This test determines your average blood sugar level during the preceding two to three months by using a formula that uses your blood samples. A1C levels of 6.5% or higher are considered to be potentially indicative of diabetes.

Random blood sugar test: Test your blood sugar at random using this test, which determines the level of glucose in your blood at any given moment. If your blood sugar level is over 200 mg/dL, it's possible that you have diabetes.

If you have any of the test findings mentioned above, your healthcare professional will most likely prescribe further testing to confirm the diagnosis of diabetes in you. It is critical to make a diabetes diagnosis and begin treatment as soon as possible in order to reduce the risk of developing diabetes-related complications.

"You have the power to take control of your diabetes, rather than letting it control you."
"Don't let diabetes hold you back. You are capable of achieving your goals and living a full, happy life."

Chapter seven

What kinds of treatments are available for diabetics?

There are many different approaches to treating diabetes, including the following:

Medication: Those who have diabetes have access to a wide variety of options when it comes to drugs that can assist in maintaining normal blood sugar levels. Insulin, oral drugs (such as metformin and sulfonylureas), and injectable therapies are all examples of these types of treatments (such as GLP-1 agonists and SGLT2 inhibitors).

Modifications to one's lifestyle: Modifications to one's lifestyle, including consuming a balanced diet, participating in regular physical activity, and learning to manage one's stress, can assist in better controlling one's blood sugar and preventing complications of diabetes.

Insulin therapy: People who have type 1 diabetes and some people who have type 2 diabetes may require insulin therapy in order to help control the levels of blood sugar in their bodies. A syringe, an insulin pen, or an insulin pump are all acceptable injection devices for insulin.

Continuous glucose monitoring (CGM): A CGM system consists of a small sensor that is placed under the skin and a handheld device that displays continuous readings of blood sugar levels. CGM systems are used by people who have diabetes. People who have diabetes may benefit from a greater understanding of how the foods they eat, the amount of physical exercise they get, and the drugs they take affect their blood sugar levels.

Education for diabetes self-management: Programs that educate persons with diabetes on how to self-manage their illness and avoid complications might be considered diabetic education for diabetes self-management. These programs may involve counseling on physical activity and stress management skills, as well as instruction on nutrition and healthy eating.

It is critical to establish a good working relationship with a healthcare professional in order to find the optimal treatment strategy for your individual requirements.

"Every day is a new opportunity to make healthy choices and manage your diabetes."

"You are strong and resilient. Don't let diabetes get in the way of living your best life."

Chapter Eight

Managing Diabetes

Alterations to one's way of life, in addition to medical treatment, are necessary for diabetes management. The following is a list of some of the more general things you can do to control your diabetes:

- Adhere to a healthy diet: A healthy diet for persons with diabetes contains a substantial amount of fresh fruits and vegetables, as well as whole grains, and places restrictions on the consumption of processed and sugary foods.

- Regular physical activity can assist you in managing your blood sugar levels, reducing the likelihood that you will develop heart disease, and improving your general health and well-being.

- Be sure to take your medication exactly as directed. It is imperative that you take your medication exactly as prescribed by your medical professional, including insulin injections if they are required.

- Check your blood sugar levels on a regular basis. If you check your blood sugar levels on a regular basis, you will be able to determine how well your treatment plan is working and make any necessary adjustments.

- Seek support: If you want to be able to control your diabetes well, it can be good to have a support network consisting of family and friends. You might also find it beneficial to become a member of a support group for those with diabetes.

It is essential to design a treatment strategy that is tailored to your needs in close collaboration with the members of your healthcare team. You are able to take control of your diabetes and lead a healthy, active life by making appropriate changes to your lifestyle and receiving appropriate medical care.

"Remember that living with diabetes requires some effort and dedication, but it is possible to manage the condition and lead a full and active life. Don't let diabetes hold you back.

Take control of your health and take the necessary steps to manage your condition effectively. With determination and the right mindset, you can overcome any challenge and achieve your goals"

Chapter Nine

Complications that are caused by diabetes

Diabetes is an ongoing disorder that develops when the body is unable to control the amount of sugar (glucose) that is present in the blood effectively. Diabetes can result in a number of complications if it is not well managed, including the following:

- Diabetes puts a person at a higher risk for a number of cardiovascular diseases, including a heart attack, a stroke, and other cardiovascular complications.
- Neuropathy is a condition that can be caused by having high blood sugar levels.

This condition can cause tingling, numbness, and pain in the extremities.

- Diabetes can also cause damage to the kidneys, a condition called nephropathy, which can progress to renal disease or even kidney failure.

- Problems with the eyes Diabetes can cause damage to the blood vessels in the eyes, which can lead to a loss of vision or even blindness.

- Diabetes can lead to skin concerns, including dry, itchy skin and an increased risk of developing skin infections.

- Problems with the feet High levels of blood sugar can cause poor circulation in the feet, which can increase the risk of foot infections and amputations.

It is essential for diabetics to maintain careful control of their condition and collaborate with the members of their healthcare team in order to avoid or reduce the severity of complications. This may include performing routine checks on blood sugar levels, adhering to a balanced diet and exercise regimen, and taking medications exactly as directed.

"Don't let diabetes hold you back. You are capable of achieving your goals and living a full, happy life."

Chapter Ten

Preventing Diabetes

Choosing to live a healthier lifestyle can help lower a person's chance of having diabetes, which is a key component in diabetes prevention. Here are some tips for preventing diabetes:

- Eat well by selecting foods that are high in nutrients but low in added sugars, saturated fats, and sodium. This will help you maintain a healthy weight. Aim to consume a wide range of produce, including fruits, vegetables, whole grains, lean proteins, and healthy fats.

- Perform regular physical activity: Aim for at least 150 minutes of exercise per week at a moderate intensity or 75 minutes of exercise per week at a strong intensity. Participating in consistent physical activity can assist in the reduction of blood sugar levels and the improvement of insulin sensitivity.

- A healthy weight should be maintained since having a BMI that is above the recommended range increases the likelihood of acquiring diabetes. Your goal should be to reach and then maintain a healthy weight by following a diet that is balanced in its macronutrient composition and by engaging in regular physical exercise.

- Consume alcohol in moderation because a high alcohol intake is associated with an increased risk of developing diabetes. If you do decide to drink alcohol, make sure you do so in a responsible manner.

- Stop smoking. Smoking raises the risk of developing diabetes and can make the complications of diabetes worse. Quit smoking. If you smoke, you should seriously consider giving up the habit in order to lower your risk of developing diabetes.

- Get an adequate amount of sleep because not getting enough sleep can cause problems with controlling blood sugar and raise the chance of developing diabetes. Aim to get between 7 and 9 hours of sleep each night.

Take steps to manage your stress. Prolonged stress can affect the body's ability to regulate blood sugar, which in turn raises the chance of developing diabetes. Find and implement good coping mechanisms for managing stress, such as going for a run, practicing meditation, or consulting a mental health expert.

You can lower your risk of acquiring diabetes and improve your general health if you pay attention to the advice in this article and make an effort to lead a healthier lifestyle.

You have the power to control your diabetes, don't let it control you."

Chapter Eleven

Living with Diabetes

Although having diabetes might make day-to-day life difficult at times, it is not impossible to lead a fulfilling and active life despite having the illness. Here are some recommendations for managing diabetes:

Adhere to a healthy diet: This may require adhering to a food plan that is customized to your personal needs and contains a balance of carbohydrates, protein, and fat in the appropriate proportions. Additionally, it is essential to cut back on the amount of additional salt and sugar you consume.

Maintaining a regular exercise routine is one of the best ways to control your blood sugar levels and enhance your overall health. Aim for at least 150 minutes of activity per week at a moderately intense level, or at least 75 minutes of exercise per week at a vigorously intense level.

It is essential that you take your insulin and any other medications exactly as directed by your doctor or other healthcare professional. If you have been given a prescription for insulin or any other medication, it is your responsibility to follow that prescription exactly. Keeping your blood sugar levels within a healthy range will be easier with this assistance.

Make sure to get your blood sugar checked on a regular basis. If you monitor your blood sugar levels, you can better manage your diabetes and avoid complications. Your healthcare practitioner will provide you with recommendations regarding how frequently you should check your blood sugar as well as what range you should aim for.

Visit your primary care physician frequently. It is critical to visit your primary care physician frequently in order to have your blood sugar levels, blood pressure, and cholesterol checked. Additionally, they are able to assist you in making any necessary alterations to your treatment plan.

Get enough sleep, learn to manage stress, and stay away from tobacco and alcohol if you want to take care of your overall health in addition to managing your diabetes. This is why it's so important to take care of your overall health.

In the event that you are troubled by the prospect of living with diabetes, do not be reluctant to discuss your worries with your healthcare professional. They are able to offer you additional support and information to help you deal with your disease and manage it.

"Living with diabetes can be challenging at times, but it's important to remember that you have the power to manage your condition and lead a healthy, fulfilling life. It may take some effort and dedication, but with the right mindset and approach, you can take charge of your health and make positive changes to improve your overall well-being".

Conclusion

Diabetes is a long-term disorder that alters the way in which the body processes sugar, also known as glucose. Samantha was diagnosed with type 1 and type 2 diabetes at the age of 16. With the support of her loved ones and healthcare professionals, she learned how to manage her condition. Diabetes can be divided into two primary categories: type 1 and type 2. Type 1 diabetes develops when the immune system attacks and destroys the cells in the pancreas that are responsible for producing insulin.

Type 2 diabetes can be prevented by maintaining a healthy weight and exercising regularly.

Diabetes is characterized by a variety of symptoms that might be experienced by a person who may or may not have the condition. Insulin, a hormone that regulates blood sugar levels, is not produced in sufficient quantities in type 1 diabetes. The body tries to rid itself of excess sugar by eliminating it through urine. High blood sugar levels can impair the body's immune system, making a person more susceptible to infections.

Some individuals who have diabetes may not have any symptoms at all. Even if you don't think you have diabetes, you should still get checked and screened for it. The chance of acquiring diabetes is proportional to a person's age, and this risk rises with age. Some risk factors, such as age and genetics, are immutable. However, maintaining a healthy weight, getting regular physical activity, and eating a healthy diet can lower your risk of developing diabetes.

Diabetes may be present when the level of glucose in the blood while fasting is 126 milligrams per deciliter (mg/dL) or greater. Diabetes may also be present if the blood sugar level is over 200 mg/dL after being monitored for two hours. Diabetics have access to a wide variety of options when it comes to drugs that can assist in maintaining normal blood sugar levels. People who have diabetes may benefit from a greater understanding of how the foods they eat, amount of physical exercise and the drugs they take affect their blood glucose levels. There are many things you can do to help manage your diabetes, as well as the need for medical treatment, in addition to making changes to your lifestyle.

Diabetes is an ongoing disorder that develops when the body is unable to control the amount of sugar (glucose) present in the blood effectively. Diabetes can result in a number of complications if it is not well managed, including nerve and eye damage and infections. Choose foods high in nutrients but low in added sugars, saturated fats, and sodium. Maintain a healthy weight by following a diet that is balanced in its macronutrient composition. Get an adequate amount of sleep because not getting enough sleep can cause problems with controlling blood sugar.

Having diabetes can be difficult but it is not impossible to lead a fulfilling and active life despite having the illness. Here are some recommendations for managing diabetes, which include adhering to a healthy diet and maintaining a regular exercise routine. Aim for at least 150 minutes of activity per week at a moderately intense level or 75 minutes of exercise at a vigorously intense level. Get enough sleep, learn to manage stress, and stay away from tobacco and alcohol if you want to take care of your overall health. It is possible to have a full and active life despite having the condition. Important steps in the management of diabetes include maintaining a healthy diet, engaging in regular physical activity and consulting a medical professional on a regular basis.

Advice

If you have diabetes, it is important to manage your blood sugar levels to avoid complications such as heart disease, stroke, nerve damage, kidney disease, and vision loss. Here are some tips for managing and living with diabetes:

Follow a healthy diet: Eat a variety of whole foods, including fruits, vegetab.les, whole grains, and lean proteins. Limit your intake of sugary drinks and snacks, and avoid processed and high-fat foods.

Get regular physical activity: Aim for at least 30 minutes of moderate-intensity exercise most days of the week. Physical activity can help lower your blood sugar levels and improve your overall health.

Take your medications as prescribed: If you are taking insulin or other medications to manage your blood sugar levels, it is important to take them as directed by your healthcare provider.

Monitor your blood sugar levels: Use a blood glucose monitor to check your blood sugar levels regularly. This will help you and your healthcare provider understand how your blood sugar levels are responding to your treatment plan.

Communicate with your healthcare team: Work with your healthcare provider and other members of your diabetes care team to create a treatment plan that works for you. Be sure to share any concerns or questions you have about your diabetes management.

By following these tips and working closely with your healthcare team, you can successfully manage your diabetes and live a healthy, active life.

Message To You

As a person with diabetes, it's important to remember that you have the strength and determination to manage your condition and live a healthy, fulfilling life. It may not always be easy, but with the right mindset and support, you can overcome any challenges that come your way. Here are a few things to remember:

You are not alone. There are many others who are living with diabetes and facing similar challenges. You can seek out support from loved ones, healthcare professionals, or online communities to help you navigate this journey.

You are in control. Although diabetes is a chronic condition, you have the power to make healthy choices that can positively impact your blood sugar levels and overall health. This includes following your treatment plan, exercising regularly, and eating a balanced diet.

Don't be too hard on yourself. It's natural to have ups and downs, and it's okay to make mistakes. What's important is that you keep trying and continue to work towards your goals.

Remember, you have the strength and resilience to manage your diabetes and live a healthy, fulfilling life. Keep moving forward and never give up!

Motivational quotes

Here are a few motivational quotes that may be helpful for people with diabetes:

"Diabetes does not define who I am, it is just a small part of my journey."

"I have diabetes, but diabetes does not have me."

"I am in control of my diabetes, not the other way around."

"I am stronger than my diabetes, and I will not let it hold me back."

"I am determined to live a healthy and active life with diabetes."

"I will not let diabetes stand in the way of my dreams and goals."

"I am committed to taking care of myself and managing my diabetes."

"I will not let diabetes define my limitations, I will define my own."

"I am grateful for the opportunity to learn and grow through my experiences with diabetes."

"I am more than my diabetes, and I will thrive despite it."

I hope these quotes inspire and motivate you to take control of your diabetes and live a healthy, happy life. Remember, you are not alone and there is support available to help you manage your diabetes effectively.